Amer A. Taqa, Nadira Hatim, Nashwah Azeez

AF152475

Natural Stain as a Substitute of Synthetic Stain

Document Nr. V209689

Amer A. Taqa, Nadira Hatim, Nashwah Azeez

Natural Stain as a Substitute of Synthetic Stain

GRIN Verlag

Die Deutsche Bibliothek verzeichnet diese Publikation in der Deutschen Nationalbibliografie; detaillierte bibliografische Daten sind im Internet über http://dnb.d-nb.de/ abrufbar.

1. Auflage 2012
Copyright © 2012 GRIN Verlag GmbH
http://www.grin.com
Druck und Bindung: Books on Demand GmbH, Norderstedt Germany
ISBN 978-3-656-37561-6

Natural Stain as a Substitute of Synthetic Stain

Nashwah S Azeez

Department of Prosthetic Dentistry

BDS, College of Dentistry, University of Mosul

Nadira A Hatim

Department of Prosthetic Dentistry

BDS, Msc (Professor) College of Dentistry, University of Mosul

Amer A Taqa

Department of Dental Basic science

Bsc, Msc, PhD (Professor) College of Dentistry, University of Mosul

ABSTRACT

Background and Objectives: Polymethyl methacrylate (PMMA) is currently the material of choice for denture base fabrication, that it has the advantages of good pigment wettability, high gloss and so on.

Uses of natural stains (amaranth and vanilla) cheap and available in our country instead of the synthetic stains with heat cure acrylic resin denture base material for matching with natural human gingiva. **Materials and Methods:** Ninety samples were prepared of pink heat cure acrylic resin Vertex[TM] material, fifteen samples with natural additives and seventy five samples with synthetic Vertex acrylic stain[TM]. The color of samples and gingival color of 24 healthy young participate were measured by Vita Easyshade device then compared between them. Statistical analysis was done by special designed program prepared for this study in Mat lab program 2010 that calculate the color difference between all the measurements that appeared only the (ΔE) that ≤ 6.8. **Results:** Results showed that (ΔE) ≤ 6.8 between some of natural and synthetic stains matched in relation to color of patients' gingiva, and some natural stains matched the color of the patients' gingiva. **Conclusions:** The results approved can be using the natural stains vanilla and amaranth instead of the synthetic Vertex acrylic stains that is clinically acceptable compared in relation to patients.

Key Words: Natural stains, Vanilla, Amaranth, PMMA.

INTRODUCTION

Polymethyl methacrylate (PMMA) is currently the material of choice for denture base fabrication [1], that it has the advantages of good pigment wettability, high gloss and so on [2].

In order to obtain a natural looking restoration, there are two crucial steps in everyday dental practice; the selection of color through shade guide which will harmoniously integrate itself with surrounding biological tissue and consequently the correct reproduction of the color in the prosthesis[3]. Healthy gingival color ranges from pale pink and pink to dark red or purple [4].

Esthetic effects are sometimes produced in a restorative material by the incorporation of colored pigments; is pigments in non metallic materials such as resin, composites, dentures acrylics, silicone maxillofacial materials and dental ceramics[5].

Synthetic stains are mainly chemical products, which have some toxicity[6]. The obtainment of coloring matter based on natural products is of considerable importance since the United States have banned the use of synthetic coloring in foods[7].

Grain Amaranth (Amaranthus paniculatus) [8] it is a natural stain that the anthocyannin is the reddish pigments in amaranth flour and vegetation appear to have great potential as a source of natural, non–toxic red dyes, this pigment is used in food industry [9].

Natural vanillin (4-hydroxy-3-methoxybenzaldehyde) is one of the most common flavor chemicals and is used in a broad range of flavors[10,11] it is a tropical orchid belonging to the family Orchidaceae [11].

Color difference (ΔE) as value for color differences became a critical in color science as well as in industries ranging from textiles to dentistry that calculated as following [12]:

$$\Delta E = [(\Delta L^*)^{2} + (\Delta a^*)^2 + (\Delta b^*)^2]^{1/2}$$

$$\Delta E = [(L^*_2 - L^*_1)^{2} + (a^*_2 - a^*_1)^2 + (b^*_2 - b^*_1)^2]^{1/2}$$

Vita EasyShade device is one that used For spectrophotometer measurement, this instrument provide data obtained over the range of visible wavelengths about 400 to 700 nm, captures the tristimuli HCL and subsequently calculates the values of L*, a* & b*[13].

MATERIALS AND METHODS

One type of pink heat-cured acrylic resin denture base material Vertex ™ type was used with natural (amaranth and vanilla), and synthetic stain ™ additives. The samples were prepared follow the recommended manufacturers' instruction powder/ liquid ratio. Curing was carried out by using conventional water bath methods in which placing flask in a thermostatically controlled water bath for curing cycle 1.5 hours at 74°C followed by 30 minutes at 100°C [14]. All prepared samples were stored in distilled water at 37°C for 7 days for conditioning before testing. Ten samples were prepared to the uniform size in dimension (30x20x1.5)

±0.03 mm (length, width and thickness respectively) [15], samples were divided into two groups:

First Group: Fifteen samples of natural stain additives type as follows:

1. Five samples with amaranth stain 0.1% wt/wt.
2. Five samples with vanilla additives 10% wt/wt.
3. Five samples with mixture of amaranth 0.02% and vanilla 0.08% respectively wt/wt.

Second Group: Seventy five samples prepared with synthetic stain [TM] additive types:

1. Fifteen samples of vertex acrylic stain [TM] no.210 (1%, 5%, and 10% wt/wt).
2. Fifteen samples of vertex acrylic stain [TM] no.220 (1%, 5%, and 10% wt/wt).
3. Fifteen samples of vertex acrylic stain [TM] no.230 (1%, 5%, and 10% wt/wt).
4. Fifteen samples of vertex acrylic stain [TM] no.240 (1%, 5%, and 10% wt/wt).
5. Fifteen samples of vertex acrylic stain [TM] no.250 (1%, 5%, and 10% wt/wt) as in Figure (1).

Color measurements were repeated five times for each sample and the mean of L*,a* and b* were calculated. Twenty four male (12) and female (12) dental students with age range 24±1 year. Mean of three

measurements of gingival color was evaluated in the anterior region (in midpoint between free gingiva and deepest point of sulcus in central and lateral incisor regions) as in Figure (2).

Measurement color matching: (CIE L*a*b*) color difference metrics were used for the performance analysis. Measurements were done by Vita Easyshade device that showed in Figure (3) to obtain the baseline L*, a*, b* values. The information from Dr.- lng. Wolfgang Rauh , a director Business Unit – Dental Devices in VITA company "can be use Easyshade to compare different samples of resins just be comparing the reported values but that the values will not correspond to values provided by other devices and similar to resins it be possible to use it to compare different gingiva but the values will not be absolute values")[16]. The total color change (ΔE) between values was calculated for each pairs evaluated using the formula:

$$\Delta E = [(\Delta L^*)^2 + (\Delta a^*)^2 + (\Delta b^*)^2]^{1/2}$$
$$\Delta E = [(L^*2 - L^*1)^2 + (a^*2 - a^*1)^2 + (b^*2 - b^*1)^2]^{1/2}$$

In principle, when $\Delta E \leq 3.7$[17] the difference in color between the paired values matched are acceptable in vitro and when $\Delta E \leq 6.8$[17] the difference in color between the paired values matched are acceptable in vivo, so the two samples are nearly have same color in vivo, when color difference be detected is > 6.8 that is not acceptable and the paired samples are not matched in vivo.

Statistical analysis carried out using a special program designed in Matlab 2010 program for this study to calculate (ΔE) between every value with all others and output appears only the paired that have (ΔE) $\leq$ 6.8.

RESULTS

The three values (L*a*b*) of the color measuring of all the prepared samples are listed in Table (1). The value of the color measurement of gingival part of the oral cavity of patients are listed in Table (2). Table (3) listed the color differences between the color of the prepared samples and the color measurement of gingival part of the oral cavity of patients.

DISCUSSIONS

Results from the Table (1) and (2) show that (ΔE) of the patient versus prepared samples with natural stain vanilla additives in 10% is acceptable and the (ΔE) of the patient versus samples with synthetic stain no. 240 in 10% was also acceptable so the natural stain vanilla could be used instead of the synthetic stain no.240.

The color of the patients gingiva was matched the color of the (prepared samples with combined both amaranth 0.01% and vanilla 0.09%) and (prepared samples with amaranth stain 0.1% additives stain) as listed in Table (3), so it could be applied in clinical uses.

Synthetic stain^{TM} no.250 in 1% with synthetic stain^{TM} no.250 in 5% and synthetic stain^{TM} no.230 in 5% with synthetic stain^{TM} no.230 in 10%

matched the same patient gingival color so increase the stain percentage from 1% to 5% and from 5% to 10% not causing a significant color changes that should increase the percentages of the stain to cause additional color and this is a waste of the material and consequence higher the cost.

Amaranth has been used for millennia to color everything to the rouge painted cheeks of South African women as it is red dyes[18], it used in dental field as additive to the dental wax[19]. Vanilla uses are mainly focused on uses in food industries, also it one commonly used remedy that has widely been reported to soothe toothaches when pain killers[20], and incorporated in the mouth rinse[21], but it's uses in dental field are not widely. Amaranth and vanilla stain are cheap and available in my country. This is a recent study of these natural stains (amaranth and vanilla) added to heat cure acrylic resin denture base as coloring agents and there is no similar previous study.

CONCLUSIONS

The results appeared that it can be using the natural stain (vanilla 10% wt/wt and amaranth 0.1% wt/wt) instead of the synthetic Vertex[TM] acrylic stain compared in relation to patients that the color difference were evaluated with(CIE L*a*b*) system. The results appeared that ΔE between tested values is ≤ 6.8 that is matched clinically.

REFERENCES

1. Mohamed S, AL-Jadi A and Ajaal T. Using of HPLC Analysis for Evaluation of Residual Monomer Content in Denture Base Material and Their Effect on Mechanical Properties. Journal of Physical Science. 2008; 19(2): 127–135.

2. Xu K, Zhou S, and Wu L. Preparation and Properties of Thermosetting Acrylic Coatings Using Titanium-oxo-cluster as a Curing Agent. Chinese Journal of Polymer Science. 2009; 27(3): 351−358.

3. Corciolani G. Study of dental color matching, color selection and color reproduction. PhD thesis 11th 2009 University of Siena, Italy.

4. Jahangiri L, Reinhardt SB, Mehra RV and Matheson PB. Relationship between tooth shade value and skin color: an observational study. J Prosthet Dent. 2002; 87(2):149-52.

5. Power J and Sakaguchi R. Graig's Restorative Dental Material.12th edition 2006; Pp:31–33.

6. Qing C, ping S, Ya-min W, Jun W, Bai-lin W and Tuo Z. Quantitative Prediction of Synthetic Food Colors by Fluorescence Spectroscopy and Radial Basis Function Neural Networks. Second International Conference on Information and Computing Science. 2009; 17–20.

7. Scoles G, Pattacini S and Covas G. Separation of the Pigment of an Amaranth , Molecules. 2000; (5)566–567.

8. Punita A and Chaturvedi A. Effect of feeding crude red palm oil (Elaeis guineensis) and grain amaranth (Amaranthus paniculatus) to hens on total lipids, cholesterol, PUFA levels and acceptability of eggs. Plant Foods for Human Nutrition. 2000; 55: 147–157.

9. Myers R. Grain Amaranth: A lost Crop of the Americas. Jefferon Institute, Columbia, MO. 2002; Pp:1–4.

10. Hagedorn S and Kaphammer B. Microbial biocatalysis in the generation of favor and fragrance chemicals. Ann Rev. Microbiol. 1994; 48:773–800.

11. Krings U and Berger R. Biotechnological production of favors and fragrances. Appl Microbiol Biotechnol .1998; 49:1–8.

12. Baltzer A and Jinoian V. The Determination of the Tooth Colors. Quintessenz Zahntechnik. 2004; 30(7):726-740.

13. Caneppele T and Torres C. Influence of surfactants on the effectiveness of bleaching gels. Clin Oral Invest. 2011; 15:57–64.

14. Hersek N , Canay S and Uzun G. Color stability of denture base acrylic resin in three food colorants . J Prosthet Dent. 1999 ;(81) 4: 375–379 .

15. Hatim N, Taqa A, Hasan R. Evaluation of the effect of curing techniques on color property of acrylic resins. Al – Rafidain Dent J. 2004; 4(1): 28–33.

16. Rauh W. VITA easyshade device. www.vita-zahnfabrik.com.

17. Johnston W and Kao E. Assessment of Appearance Match by Visual Observation and Clinical Colorimetry. J Dent Res. 1989; 68:819–822.

18. Jonnalagadda P, Rao P, Bhat R and Nadu A. Type, Extent and Use of Colors in Ready to Eat (RTE) Foods Prepared in the non Industrial Sector- Case Study from Hyderabad, India. International journal of food science and technology. 2004; 39(2):125–131.

.

19. Alubaidi AW. Prosthetic applicaton of experimental modeling wax with some additives. (2008): MSc Thesis; College of Dentistry / University of Mosul.

20. www. Vanilla- toothaches.com

21. Al-Sandook TA . Efficacy of Vanillin as a principle Constituent in mouth rinse. Iraqi Dent J. 1998; 23: 5-12.

Table (1): L, a and b, Mean of Three Values of the Prepared Samples
with Natural and Synthetic Stain Additives.

Prepared samples	L	a	B
P V (10 %)	53.44	27.28	12.04
P A (0.1 %)	41.6	35.58	15.3
P 9.9+ A 0.01 + v0.09 (1%)	42.16	38.26	17.7
P $_{st1}$ (1 %)	51.78	29.92	11.92
P $_{st2}$ (1 %)	52.08	29.86	11.28
P $_{st3}$ (1 %)	51.9	30.22	11.4
P $_{st4}$ (1 %)	54	30.26	13.12
P $_{st5}$ (1 %)	49.12	27.32	10.84
P $_{st1}$ (5 %)	54.1	28.26	11.06
P $_{st2}$ (5 %)	57.16	28.02	12.06
P $_{st3}$ (5 %)	53.9	30.92	12.72
P $_{st4}$ (5 %)	53.84	33.04	13.9
P $_{st5}$ (5 %)	43.78	24.14	11.74
P $_{St1}$ (10 %)	55.2	25.7	10.06
P $_{St2}$ (10 %)	57.16	26.86	11
P $_{St3}$ (10 %)	55.12	30.42	14.04
P $_{St4}$ (10 %)	49.94	31.68	12.92
P $_{St5}$ (10 %)	44.02	18.78	12.84

L=lightness, a=redness and greenness, b=yellowness and blueness, P=pink acrylic
powder, v=vanilla, A=amaranth, $_{st1-5}$= synthetic stain no.210–250.

Table (2): The Mean Values of Color Measuring of the Patient's Gingiva.

patients	Gender	Area	L	a	b
1	f	Region a	58.2	19.5	25.6
1	f	Region b	53.7	28.0	27.0
2	f	Region a	50.8	27.2	21.6
2	f	Region b	59.7	27.6	26.9
3	f	Region a	38.9	26.7	25.3
3	f	Region b	44.2	25.1	29.6
4	f	Region a	57.5	16.5	25.6
4	f	Region b	67.0	10.6	28.3
5	f	Region a	64.7	10.2	25.9
5	f	Region b	45.4	29.1	19.3
6	f	Region a	76.2	3.0	25.8
6	f	Region b	50.4	26.7	15.2
7	f	Region a	52.9	19.0	23.8
7	f	Region b	48.9	23.2	13.6
8	f	Region a	69.5	7.2	50.1
8	f	Region b	5.8	19.8	28.4
9	f	Region a	50.8	17.1	25.3
9	f	Region b	51.7	17.6	36.3
10	f	Region a	52.9	16.3	21.8
10	f	Region b	55.0	19.5	31.9
11	f	Region a	47.4	25.2	21.7
11	f	Region b	55.6	16.2	38.5
12	f	Region a	53.5	24.1	28.0

12	f	Region b	71.0	12.9	31.6
13	m	Region a	42.6	36.0	20.2
13	m	Region b	57.2	14.8	27.2
14	m	Region a	59.3	16.7	23.5
14	m	Region b	53.7	25.8	24.8
15	m	Region a	40.2	33.7	17.8
15	m	Region b	54.4	22.7	24.7
16	m	Region a	61.7	16.0	28.7
16	m	Region b	46.2	31.6	21.3
17	m	Region a	56.9	17.1	28.4
17	m	Region b	63.4	15.5	29.6
18	m	Region a	66.0	12.1	31.2
18	m	Region b	54.7	22.4	24.2
19	m	Region a	60.4	15.2	35.5
19	m	Region b	55.1	15.2	35.5
20	m	Region a	58.6	16.3	25.9
20	m	Region b	52.4	26.5	22.4
21	m	Region a	54.8	19.1	28.8
21	m	Region b	57.2	15.2	27.2
22	m	Region a	74.0	6.6	34.9
22	m	Region b	60.5	16.6	28.2
23	m	Region a	53.8	22.4	30.4
23	m	Region b	57.2	17.3	36.8
24	m	Region a	52.3	20.7	25.5
24	m	Region b	57.3	18.2	29.6

L=degree of lightness, a=degree of redness and greenness, b=degree of yellowness and blueness, m=male, f=female, region a= central incisor region, region b = lateral incisor region.

Table (3): (ΔE) of the Samples that is ≤ 6.8.

Compared values	ΔE
13ma v P 9.9 + A 0.01 + v0.09 (1 %)	3.398706
15ma v P A (0.1 %)	3.42701
6fb v P V (10 %)	4.423076
6fb v P st5 (1 %)	4.586109
6fb v P st1 (1 %)	4.799083
7fb v P st5 (1 %)	4.96391
6fb v P St4 (10 %)	5.496399
7fb v P st5 (5 %)	5.527893
6fb v P st3 (5 %)	6.017375
6fb v P st3 (10 %)	6.120654

L=lightness, a=redness and greenness, b=yellowness and blueness.

P=pink acrylic powder, v=vanilla, A=amaranth, st_{1-5} = synthetic stain no.210-250, 1–15=patients.

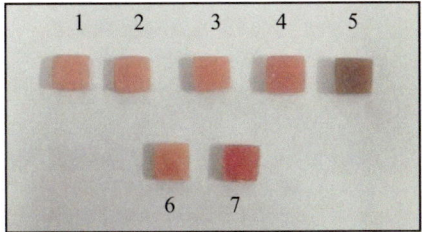

(1): Samples with synthetic stain No.210 additives, (2): Samples with synthetic stain No.220 additives, (3): Samples with synthetic stain No.230 additives (4): Samples with synthetic stain No.240 additives (5): Samples with synthetic stain No.250 additives, (6): Samples with vanilla additives and (7): Samples with amaranth additives.

Figure (1): Samples of synthetic and natural stain additives.

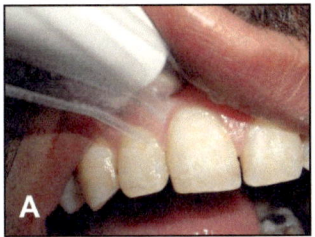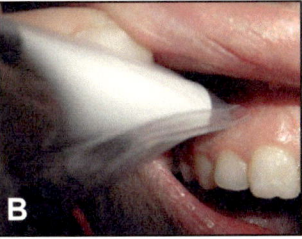

Figure (2): Measuring gingival color at (A); Central incisor region, (B); Lateral incisor region.

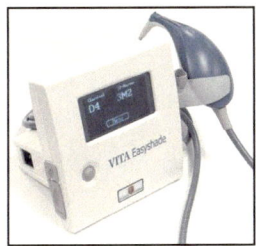

Figure (3) Easyshade device.